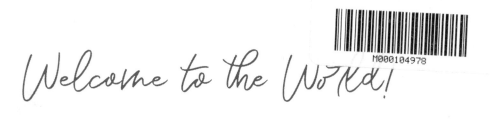

_____
_____
_____

BORN ON:

_____

@

_____

Height: _____

Weight: _____

Date:_____

NOTES FROM ROUNDS:

FEEDINGS:

VITALS/WEIGHTS:

TESTS/XRAYS/PROCEDURES:

DAILY MILESTONES:

QUESTIONS FOR DOCTORS/NURSES:

GOALS:

BUMPS IN THE ROAD:

VISITOR LOG & MEMORIES:

Date: _____

NOTES FROM ROUNDS:

FEEDINGS:

VITALS/WEIGHTS:

TESTS/XRAYS/PROCEDURES:

DAILY MILESTONES:

QUESTIONS FOR
DOCTORS/NURSES:

GOALS:

BUMPS IN THE ROAD:

VISITOR LOG & MEMORIES:

Date:_____

NOTES FROM ROUNDS:

FEEDINGS:

VITALS/WEIGHTS:

TESTS/XRAYS/PROCEDURES:

DAILY MILESTONES:

QUESTIONS FOR
DOCTORS/NURSES:

GOALS:

BUMPS IN THE ROAD:

VISITOR LOG & MEMORIES:

Date:_____

NOTES FROM ROUNDS:

FEEDINGS:

VITALS/WEIGHTS:

TESTS/XRAYS/PROCEDURES:

DAILY MILESTONES:

QUESTIONS FOR
DOCTORS/NURSES:

GOALS:

BUMPS IN THE ROAD:

VISITOR LOG & MEMORIES:

Date: _____

NOTES FROM ROUNDS:

FEEDINGS:

VITALS/WEIGHTS:

TESTS/XRAYS/PROCEDURES:

DAILY MILESTONES:

QUESTIONS FOR
DOCTORS/NURSES:

GOALS:

BUMPS IN THE ROAD:

VISITOR LOG & MEMORIES:

Date: _____

NOTES FROM ROUNDS:

FEEDINGS:

VITALS/WEIGHTS:

TESTS/XRAYS/PROCEDURES:

DAILY MILESTONES:

QUESTIONS FOR DOCTORS/NURSES:

GOALS:

BUMPS IN THE ROAD:

VISITOR LOG & MEMORIES:

Date:_____

NOTES FROM ROUNDS:

FEEDINGS:

VITALS/WEIGHTS:

TESTS/XRAYS/PROCEDURES:

DAILY MILESTONES:

QUESTIONS FOR DOCTORS/NURSES:

GOALS:

BUMPS IN THE ROAD:

VISITOR LOG & MEMORIES:

Date: _____

NOTES FROM ROUNDS:

FEEDINGS:

VITALS/WEIGHTS:

TESTS/XRAYS/PROCEDURES:

DAILY MILESTONES:

QUESTIONS FOR
DOCTORS/NURSES:

GOALS:

BUMPS IN THE ROAD:

VISITOR LOG & MEMORIES:

Date: _____

NOTES FROM ROUNDS:

FEEDINGS:

VITALS/WEIGHTS:

TESTS/XRAYS/PROCEDURES:

DAILY MILESTONES:

QUESTIONS FOR
DOCTORS/NURSES:

GOALS:

BUMPS IN THE ROAD:

VISITOR LOG & MEMORIES:

Date: _____

NOTES FROM ROUNDS:

FEEDINGS:

VITALS/WEIGHTS:

TESTS/XRAYS/PROCEDURES:

DAILY MILESTONES:

QUESTIONS FOR
DOCTORS/NURSES:

GOALS:

BUMPS IN THE ROAD:

VISITOR LOG & MEMORIES:

Date: _____

NOTES FROM
ROUNDS:

FEEDINGS:

VITALS/WEIGHTS:

TESTS/XRAYS/PROCEDURES:

DAILY MILESTONES:

QUESTIONS FOR
DOCTORS/NURSES:

GOALS:

BUMPS IN THE ROAD:

VISITOR LOG & MEMORIES:

Date: _____

NOTES FROM ROUNDS:

FEEDINGS:

VITALS/WEIGHTS:

TESTS/XRAYS/PROCEDURES:

DAILY MILESTONES:

QUESTIONS FOR
DOCTORS/NURSES:

GOALS:

BUMPS IN THE ROAD:

VISITOR LOG & MEMORIES:

Date: _____

NOTES FROM ROUNDS:

FEEDINGS:

VITALS/WEIGHTS:

TESTS/XRAYS/PROCEDURES:

DAILY MILESTONES:

QUESTIONS FOR DOCTORS/NURSES:

GOALS:

BUMPS IN THE ROAD:

VISITOR LOG & MEMORIES:

Date:_____

NOTES FROM ROUNDS:

FEEDINGS:

VITALS/WEIGHTS:

TESTS/XRAYS/PROCEDURES:

DAILY MILESTONES:

QUESTIONS FOR
DOCTORS/NURSES:

GOALS:

BUMPS IN THE ROAD:

VISITOR LOG & MEMORIES:

Date:_____

NOTES FROM ROUNDS:

FEEDINGS:

VITALS/WEIGHTS:

TESTS/XRAYS/PROCEDURES:

DAILY MILESTONES:

QUESTIONS FOR
DOCTORS/NURSES:

GOALS:

BUMPS IN THE ROAD:

VISITOR LOG & MEMORIES:

Date: _____

NOTES FROM ROUNDS:

FEEDINGS:

VITALS/WEIGHTS:

TESTS/XRAYS/PROCEDURES:

DAILY MILESTONES:

QUESTIONS FOR
DOCTORS/NURSES:

GOALS:

BUMPS IN THE ROAD:

VISITOR LOG & MEMORIES:

Date:_____

NOTES FROM ROUNDS:

FEEDINGS:

VITALS/WEIGHTS:

TESTS/XRAYS/PROCEDURES:

DAILY MILESTONES:

QUESTIONS FOR
DOCTORS/NURSES:

GOALS:

BUMPS IN THE ROAD:

VISITOR LOG & MEMORIES:

Date:_____

NOTES FROM ROUNDS:

FEEDINGS:

VITALS/WEIGHTS:

TESTS/XRAYS/PROCEDURES:

DAILY MILESTONES:

QUESTIONS FOR
DOCTORS/NURSES:

GOALS:

BUMPS IN THE ROAD:

VISITOR LOG & MEMORIES:

Date:_____

NOTES FROM ROUNDS:

FEEDINGS:

VITALS/WEIGHTS:

TESTS/XRAYS/PROCEDURES:

DAILY MILESTONES:

QUESTIONS FOR
DOCTORS/NURSES:

GOALS:

BUMPS IN THE ROAD:

VISITOR LOG & MEMORIES:

Date: _____

NOTES FROM ROUNDS:

FEEDINGS:

VITALS/WEIGHTS:

TESTS/XRAYS/PROCEDURES:

DAILY MILESTONES:

QUESTIONS FOR
DOCTORS/NURSES:

GOALS:

BUMPS IN THE ROAD:

VISITOR LOG & MEMORIES:

Date:_____

NOTES FROM ROUNDS:

FEEDINGS:

VITALS/WEIGHTS:

TESTS/XRAYS/PROCEDURES:

DAILY MILESTONES:

QUESTIONS FOR DOCTORS/NURSES:

GOALS:

BUMPS IN THE ROAD:

VISITOR LOG & MEMORIES:

Date:_____

NOTES FROM ROUNDS:

FEEDINGS:

VITALS/WEIGHTS:

TESTS/XRAYS/PROCEDURES:

DAILY MILESTONES:

QUESTIONS FOR
DOCTORS/NURSES:

GOALS:

BUMPS IN THE ROAD:

VISITOR LOG & MEMORIES:

Date:_____

NOTES FROM ROUNDS:

FEEDINGS:

VITALS/WEIGHTS:

TESTS/XRAYS/PROCEDURES:

DAILY MILESTONES:

QUESTIONS FOR
DOCTORS/NURSES:

GOALS:

BUMPS IN THE ROAD:

VISITOR LOG & MEMORIES:

Date: _____

NOTES FROM ROUNDS:

FEEDINGS:

VITALS/WEIGHTS:

TESTS/XRAYS/PROCEDURES:

DAILY MILESTONES:

QUESTIONS FOR
DOCTORS/NURSES:

GOALS:

BUMPS IN THE ROAD:

VISITOR LOG & MEMORIES:

Date:_____

NOTES FROM ROUNDS:

FEEDINGS:

VITALS/WEIGHTS:

TESTS/XRAYS/PROCEDURES:

DAILY MILESTONES:

QUESTIONS FOR
DOCTORS/NURSES:

GOALS:

BUMPS IN THE ROAD:

VISITOR LOG & MEMORIES:

Date:_____

NOTES FROM ROUNDS:

FEEDINGS:

VITALS/WEIGHTS:

TESTS/XRAYS/PROCEDURES:

DAILY MILESTONES:

QUESTIONS FOR
DOCTORS/NURSES:

GOALS:

BUMPS IN THE ROAD:

VISITOR LOG & MEMORIES:

NOTES FROM ROUNDS:

FEEDINGS:

VITALS/WEIGHTS:

TESTS/XRAYS/PROCEDURES:

DAILY MILESTONES:

QUESTIONS FOR
DOCTORS/NURSES:

GOALS:

BUMPS IN THE ROAD:

VISITOR LOG & MEMORIES:

Date: _____

NOTES FROM ROUNDS:

FEEDINGS:

VITALS/WEIGHTS:

TESTS/XRAYS/PROCEDURES:

DAILY MILESTONES:

QUESTIONS FOR
DOCTORS/NURSES:

GOALS:

BUMPS IN THE ROAD:

VISITOR LOG & MEMORIES:

Date:_____

NOTES FROM
ROUNDS:

FEEDINGS:

VITALS/WEIGHTS:

TESTS/XRAYS/PROCEDURES:

DAILY MILESTONES:

QUESTIONS FOR
DOCTORS/NURSES:

GOALS:

BUMPS IN THE ROAD:

VISITOR LOG & MEMORIES:

Date:_____

NOTES FROM ROUNDS:

FEEDINGS:

VITALS/WEIGHTS:

TESTS/XRAYS/PROCEDURES:

DAILY MILESTONES:

QUESTIONS FOR
DOCTORS/NURSES:

GOALS:

BUMPS IN THE ROAD:

VISITOR LOG & MEMORIES:

Date: _____

NOTES FROM ROUNDS:

FEEDINGS:

VITALS/WEIGHTS:

TESTS/XRAYS/PROCEDURES:

DAILY MILESTONES:

QUESTIONS FOR DOCTORS/NURSES:

GOALS:

BUMPS IN THE ROAD:

VISITOR LOG & MEMORIES:

Date: _____

NOTES FROM ROUNDS:

FEEDINGS:

VITALS/WEIGHTS:

TESTS/XRAYS/PROCEDURES:

DAILY MILESTONES:

QUESTIONS FOR
DOCTORS/NURSES:

GOALS:

BUMPS IN THE ROAD:

VISITOR LOG & MEMORIES:

Date:_____

NOTES FROM ROUNDS:

FEEDINGS:

VITALS/WEIGHTS:

TESTS/XRAYS/PROCEDURES:

DAILY MILESTONES:

QUESTIONS FOR DOCTORS/NURSES:

GOALS:

BUMPS IN THE ROAD:

VISITOR LOG & MEMORIES:

Date: _____

NOTES FROM ROUNDS:

FEEDINGS:

VITALS/WEIGHTS:

TESTS/XRAYS/PROCEDURES:

DAILY MILESTONES:

QUESTIONS FOR
DOCTORS/NURSES:

GOALS:

BUMPS IN THE ROAD:

VISITOR LOG & MEMORIES:

Date: _____

NOTES FROM ROUNDS:

FEEDINGS:

VITALS/WEIGHTS:

TESTS/XRAYS/PROCEDURES:

DAILY MILESTONES:

QUESTIONS FOR DOCTORS/NURSES:

GOALS:

BUMPS IN THE ROAD:

VISITOR LOG & MEMORIES:

Date:_____

NOTES FROM ROUNDS:

FEEDINGS:

VITALS/WEIGHTS:

TESTS/XRAYS/PROCEDURES:

DAILY MILESTONES:

QUESTIONS FOR
DOCTORS/NURSES:

GOALS:

BUMPS IN THE ROAD:

VISITOR LOG & MEMORIES:

Date: _____

NOTES FROM ROUNDS:

FEEDINGS:

VITALS/WEIGHTS:

TESTS/XRAYS/PROCEDURES:

DAILY MILESTONES:

QUESTIONS FOR
DOCTORS/NURSES:

GOALS:

BUMPS IN THE ROAD:

VISITOR LOG & MEMORIES:

Date: _____

NOTES FROM ROUNDS:

FEEDINGS:

VITALS/WEIGHTS:

TESTS/XRAYS/PROCEDURES:

DAILY MILESTONES:

QUESTIONS FOR DOCTORS/NURSES:

GOALS:

BUMPS IN THE ROAD:

VISITOR LOG & MEMORIES:

NOTES FROM ROUNDS:

FEEDINGS:

VITALS/WEIGHTS:

TESTS/XRAYS/PROCEDURES:

DAILY MILESTONES:

QUESTIONS FOR
DOCTORS/NURSES:

GOALS:

BUMPS IN THE ROAD:

VISITOR LOG & MEMORIES:

Date: _____

NOTES FROM ROUNDS:

FEEDINGS:

VITALS/WEIGHTS:

TESTS/XRAYS/PROCEDURES:

DAILY MILESTONES:

QUESTIONS FOR
DOCTORS/NURSES:

GOALS:

BUMPS IN THE ROAD:

VISITOR LOG & MEMORIES:

Date:_____

NOTES FROM
ROUNDS:

FEEDINGS:

VITALS/WEIGHTS:

TESTS/XRAYS/PROCEDURES:

DAILY MILESTONES:

QUESTIONS FOR
DOCTORS/NURSES:

GOALS:

BUMPS IN THE ROAD:

VISITOR LOG & MEMORIES:

Date:_____

NOTES FROM ROUNDS:

FEEDINGS:

VITALS/WEIGHTS:

TESTS/XRAYS/PROCEDURES:

DAILY MILESTONES:

QUESTIONS FOR
DOCTORS/NURSES:

GOALS:

BUMPS IN THE ROAD:

VISITOR LOG & MEMORIES:

Date: _____

NOTES FROM ROUNDS:

FEEDINGS:

VITALS/WEIGHTS:

TESTS/XRAYS/PROCEDURES:

DAILY MILESTONES:

QUESTIONS FOR DOCTORS/NURSES:

GOALS:

BUMPS IN THE ROAD:

VISITOR LOG & MEMORIES:

NOTES FROM ROUNDS:

FEEDINGS:

VITALS/WEIGHTS:

TESTS/XRAYS/PROCEDURES:

DAILY MILESTONES:

QUESTIONS FOR
DOCTORS/NURSES:

GOALS:

BUMPS IN THE ROAD:

VISITOR LOG & MEMORIES:

Date: _____

NOTES FROM ROUNDS:

FEEDINGS:

VITALS/WEIGHTS:

TESTS/XRAYS/PROCEDURES:

DAILY MILESTONES:

QUESTIONS FOR
DOCTORS/NURSES:

GOALS:

BUMPS IN THE ROAD:

VISITOR LOG & MEMORIES:

Date:_____

NOTES FROM ROUNDS:

FEEDINGS:

VITALS/WEIGHTS:

TESTS/XRAYS/PROCEDURES:

DAILY MILESTONES:

QUESTIONS FOR
DOCTORS/NURSES:

GOALS:

BUMPS IN THE ROAD:

VISITOR LOG & MEMORIES:

Date:_____

NOTES FROM ROUNDS:

FEEDINGS:

VITALS/WEIGHTS:

TESTS/XRAYS/PROCEDURES:

DAILY MILESTONES:

QUESTIONS FOR
DOCTORS/NURSES:

GOALS:

BUMPS IN THE ROAD:

VISITOR LOG & MEMORIES:

Date: _____

NOTES FROM ROUNDS:

FEEDINGS:

VITALS/WEIGHTS:

TESTS/XRAYS/PROCEDURES:

DAILY MILESTONES:

QUESTIONS FOR
DOCTORS/NURSES:

GOALS:

BUMPS IN THE ROAD:

VISITOR LOG & MEMORIES:

Date: _____

NOTES FROM ROUNDS:

FEEDINGS:

VITALS/WEIGHTS:

TESTS/XRAYS/PROCEDURES:

DAILY MILESTONES:

QUESTIONS FOR
DOCTORS/NURSES:

GOALS:

BUMPS IN THE ROAD:

VISITOR LOG & MEMORIES:

Date: _____

NOTES FROM ROUNDS:

FEEDINGS:

VITALS/WEIGHTS:

TESTS/XRAYS/PROCEDURES:

DAILY MILESTONES:

QUESTIONS FOR
DOCTORS/NURSES:

GOALS:

BUMPS IN THE ROAD:

VISITOR LOG & MEMORIES:

Date:_____

NOTES FROM ROUNDS:

FEEDINGS:

VITALS/WEIGHTS:

TESTS/XRAYS/PROCEDURES:

DAILY MILESTONES:

QUESTIONS FOR
DOCTORS/NURSES:

GOALS:

BUMPS IN THE ROAD:

VISITOR LOG & MEMORIES:

Date:_____

NOTES FROM ROUNDS:

FEEDINGS:

VITALS/WEIGHTS:

TESTS/XRAYS/PROCEDURES:

DAILY MILESTONES:

QUESTIONS FOR
DOCTORS/NURSES:

GOALS:

BUMPS IN THE ROAD:

VISITOR LOG & MEMORIES:

Date: _____

NOTES FROM ROUNDS:

FEEDINGS:

VITALS/WEIGHTS:

TESTS/XRAYS/PROCEDURES:

DAILY MILESTONES:

QUESTIONS FOR
DOCTORS/NURSES:

GOALS:

BUMPS IN THE ROAD:

VISITOR LOG & MEMORIES:

Date:_____

NOTES FROM
ROUNDS:

FEEDINGS:

VITALS/WEIGHTS:

TESTS/XRAYS/PROCEDURES:

DAILY MILESTONES:

QUESTIONS FOR
DOCTORS/NURSES:

GOALS:

BUMPS IN THE ROAD:

VISITOR LOG & MEMORIES:

NOTES FROM ROUNDS:

FEEDINGS:

VITALS/WEIGHTS:

TESTS/XRAYS/PROCEDURES:

DAILY MILESTONES:

QUESTIONS FOR
DOCTORS/NURSES:

GOALS:

BUMPS IN THE ROAD:

VISITOR LOG & MEMORIES:

$Date:$ _____

NOTES FROM ROUNDS:

FEEDINGS:

VITALS/WEIGHTS:

TESTS/XRAYS/PROCEDURES:

DAILY MILESTONES:

QUESTIONS FOR DOCTORS/NURSES:

GOALS:

BUMPS IN THE ROAD:

VISITOR LOG & MEMORIES:

Date:_____

NOTES FROM
ROUNDS:

FEEDINGS:

VITALS/WEIGHTS:

TESTS/XRAYS/PROCEDURES:

DAILY MILESTONES:

QUESTIONS FOR
DOCTORS/NURSES:

GOALS:

BUMPS IN THE ROAD:

VISITOR LOG & MEMORIES:

Date: _____

NOTES FROM ROUNDS:

FEEDINGS:

VITALS/WEIGHTS:

TESTS/XRAYS/PROCEDURES:

DAILY MILESTONES:

QUESTIONS FOR
DOCTORS/NURSES:

GOALS:

BUMPS IN THE ROAD:

VISITOR LOG & MEMORIES:

Date:_____

NOTES FROM ROUNDS:

FEEDINGS:

VITALS/WEIGHTS:

TESTS/XRAYS/PROCEDURES:

DAILY MILESTONES:

QUESTIONS FOR
DOCTORS/NURSES:

GOALS:

BUMPS IN THE ROAD:

VISITOR LOG & MEMORIES:

Date:_____

NOTES FROM ROUNDS:

FEEDINGS:

VITALS/WEIGHTS:

TESTS/XRAYS/PROCEDURES:

DAILY MILESTONES:

QUESTIONS FOR
DOCTORS/NURSES:

GOALS:

BUMPS IN THE ROAD:

VISITOR LOG & MEMORIES:

Graduation Day!

WE BROUGHT YOU HOME:

_____

Height: _____

Weight: _____

TIME SPENT IN THE NICU:

_____

Welcome Home Child!

Made in the USA
Columbia, SC
16 April 2020